JUICING AND SMOOTHIES FOR FIBROID

1500 DAYS JUICING AND SMOOTHIE RECIPES FOR FIBROID HEALTH AND RESTORE PRODUCTIVE LIFE

KAREN EDMONDS

1

TABLE OF CONTENT

STAY
HAPPY AND
HEATHY

INTRODUCTION

In a society where wellbeing is prioritised, the goal of optimal health frequently overlaps with the effort to control disorders such as fibroids. Fibroids, which are noncancerous growths in the uterus, are a growing health issue for many women. Using the transformational power of nature's elixirs, this guide takes you on an educational voyage into the world of "Juicing and Smoothies for Fibroids." Consider vivid combinations bursting with nutrient-dense fruits, green veggies, and medicinal herbs that work together to fight the obstacles provided by fibroids.

This investigation is more than just mixing ingredients; it is a journey to discover how the creative fusion of nature's richness may provide relief and vigour. Beyond the wide range of flavours and colours lies a nutritional armament designed to reinforce the body against the effects of fibroids. Unravelling the mysteries of specific substances, we look at superfood synergy, antioxidant potency, and herbal calming qualities. Join us as we explore the possibilities of green goddess elixirs and berry-infused potions, inspiring those on a path to holistic wellbeing.

Prepare to be intrigued by the enticing possibilities of nutrition and the transformational power of modest but significant lifestyle changes. This book will help you not only manage fibroids, but also thrive in tune with your body's natural resilience. Welcome to a world where the blender becomes a source of optimism, with each drink promising a better, more vibrant existence.

CHAPTER 1: OVERVIEW OF FIBROIDS

Fibroids, noncancerous tumours that form in the uterus, have become a common health problem affecting a large number of women globally. These benign growths, also known as leiomyomas or myomas, fluctuate in size and can produce a variety of symptoms, including pelvic discomfort and heavy menstrual flow. Understanding the complexities of fibroids is critical in developing appropriate management plans.

Fibroids form inside the muscular walls of the uterus and might appear as a single growth or many. While the specific reason is unknown, hormone imbalances, genetics, and environmental influences are thought to contribute to its development. Because these growths frequently thrive on oestrogen, they are more noticeable throughout the reproductive years.

Importantly, new study emphasises the importance of food in controlling fibroids. Dietary choices can have a substantial impact on hormonal balance, inflammatory levels, and general well-being, all of which play important roles in the advancement of fibroids. This section investigates the relationship between fibroids and food, focusing on the effect of nutrition on symptom severity and the possibility for dietary changes to reduce the burden of fibroid-related difficulties.

Join us on a journey exploring the complex relationship between what we eat and how we manage fibroids, discovering the transformative power of a well-balanced and focused diet in promoting uterine health and general vigour.

Nutritional Approach to Fibroids

Fibroids, which are benign growths in the uterus, require a varied approach to treatment, and food plays an important role in their genesis and evolution. Understanding the complex interaction between nutrition and fibroids allows people to make more appropriate dietary choices that can benefit their uterine health.

Role of nutrition in Fibroid Management: Fibroid development is influenced by hormonal imbalances, which may be controlled by nutrition. Certain meals can either increase or decrease oestrogen levels, a major component in fibroid formation. Adopting a hormonally balanced diet is critical for efficiently controlling fibroids.

Nutrients for Fibroid Health: Some nutrients are essential for uterine health and may help control fibroids. Key nutrients are:

Fibre: A high-fiber diet enhances oestrogen metabolism and regular bowel movements, which aids in the disposal of excess oestrogen.

Vitamins A, C, and E: Antioxidant-rich vitamins prevent oxidative stress and inflammation, potentially alleviating fibroid symptoms.

Iron: Treating iron-deficiency anaemia caused by excessive menstrual flow due to fibroids is critical for general health.

Omega 3 Fatty Acids: These fats, which may be found in fish, flaxseeds, and walnuts, have anti-inflammatory qualities and may help with symptoms.

Foods to Include or Avoid:

Include:

Leafy Greens: High in iron and fibre, leafy greens promote general health and hormone balance.

Cruciferous vegetables: They include broccoli, kale, and Brussels sprouts, which contain chemicals that help in oestrogen metabolism.

Berries: Berries are high in antioxidants and help to counteract oxidative stress.

Fatty Fish: Omega-3 fatty acids in fish may have anti-inflammatory properties.

Whole Grains: Fiber-rich whole grains promote intestinal health.

Avoid:

Highly processed foods may include chemicals that have a harmful effect on hormone balance.

Red and processed meats: High intake may raise the risk of fibroids.

Caffeine with alcohol: Excessive use may cause hormonal disturbances.

Individuals can use nutrition to their advantage in the treatment of fibroids by eating a nutrient-dense, well-balanced diet. This complete dietary approach, when combined with other lifestyle changes, provides a proactive method for improving uterine health and general well-being.

Purpose of Juicing and Smoothies

In the pursuit of maximum health and well-being, including juicing and smoothies into one's lifestyle is more than just a trend; it is a comprehensive approach to nutrition with several advantages. These liquid concoctions, made from a variety of fresh fruits, vegetables, and health-enhancing additives, are nutrient-dense, providing a quick and pleasant method to improve one's eating habits.

Nutrient Density: Juicing and smoothies are effective methods of enhancing nutrient intake. Condensing a mix of fruits and vegetables into a single glass allows people to readily ingest a wide range of vitamins, minerals, antioxidants, and phytonutrients that promote overall health and vitality.

Digestive Ease: Juices and smoothies are easier to digest since they are liquid. Nutrients are easily absorbed, making it a gentle and efficient approach to fuel the body while minimising stress on the digestive system.

Hydration Boost: Many fruits and vegetables have a significant amount of water, which helps to keep them hydrated. Juices and smoothies provide a pleasant alternative to plain water, making it simpler for people to stay hydrated throughout the day.

Detoxification Support: Certain nutrients, such as leafy greens and citrus fruits, are well known for their detoxifying qualities. Juicing and smoothies can help promote the body's natural detoxification processes, assisting in the removal of waste and pollutants.

Convenience in Nutrition: In today's fast-paced world, juicing and smoothies offer a quick and handy approach to meet nutritional demands. These beverages are ideal for a quick breakfast, snack, or post-workout refreshing.

Tailored Health objectives: Because juicing and smoothies are versatile, they may be customised to meet specific health objectives. These beverages may be adjusted to match individual needs for improved energy, immunological support, weight control, or particular nutritional targeting.

As we dig deeper into the world of juicing and smoothies, it becomes clear that their purpose goes beyond simple refreshment; they serve as a bright entryway to a nutrient-rich, health-conscious lifestyle. These beverages provide a wonderful way to feed the body and begin on a path to optimal well-being by skillfully combining flavours and useful components.

CHAPTER 2: CHOOSING THE RIGHT INGREDIENTS

Making juice and smoothies that promote fibroid management necessitates careful component selection. By mixing nutrient-dense foods with anti-inflammatory and hormone balancing characteristics, you may create beverages that not only satisfy your taste buds but also benefit your uterine health. Here is how to choose the correct ingredients:

Fruits and Vegetables for Fibroid Health:

Berries: Blueberries, strawberries, and raspberries are high in antioxidants, which help fight oxidative stress.

Citrus fruits: such as oranges, lemons, and grapefruits contain vitamin C and bioflavonoids, which may help reduce inflammation.

Leafy Greens: Spinach, kale, and collard greens include iron and fibre, which promote general health.

Pineapple: contains bromelain, which is an enzyme with anti-inflammatory effects.

Apples: They are high in fibre and phytoestrogens, which may help regulate oestrogen levels.

Superfoods and Supplements:

Flaxseeds: High in omega-3 fatty acids and fibre, flaxseeds promote hormonal balance.

Chia seeds: Include omega-3 fatty acids, fibre, and antioxidants, which contribute to general health.

Turmeric: It is known for its anti-inflammatory qualities, can be used in powder or root form.

Ginger: It has anti-inflammatory properties and provides a zesty flavour to your beverages.

Spirulina: Is a nutrient-dense algae that may include anti-inflammatory and antioxidant properties.

The Importance of Organic Produce

Choose organic fruits and vegetables to avoid exposure to pesticides and herbicides, which can alter hormonal balance.

Incorporating these components into your juicing and smoothie recipes may result in a symphony of flavours while also encouraging fibroid-friendly nutrition. Experiment with different combinations to see what matches your taste and fits with your health goals. Remember to check with a healthcare practitioner, especially if you have specific dietary limitations or questions about your fibroid treatment plan.

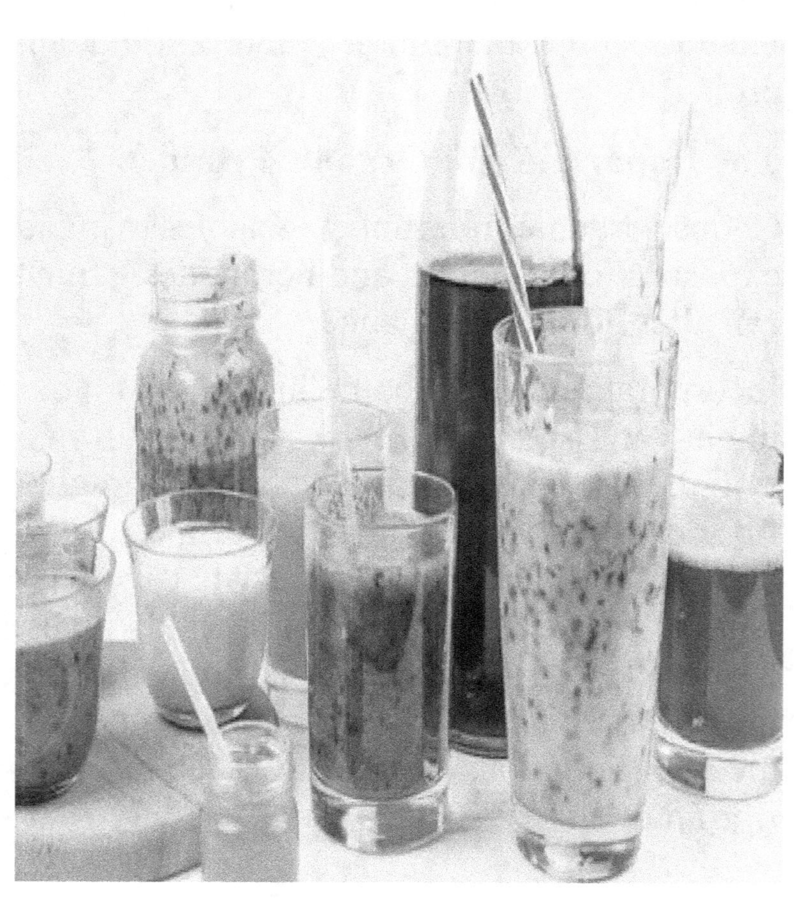

CHAPTER 3: JUICING RECIPES FOR FIBROIDS

Ingredients:

- 2 cups of kale leaves
- 1 cucumber
- 1 green apple
- 1 lemon (peeled)
- 1-inch piece of ginger
- Handful of mint leaves

Preparation:

- Wash all ingredients well.
- Cut the cucumber and green apple into eatable pieces.
- Remove the stems from the kale leaves.
- Peel the lemons and ginger.
- Run kale, cucumber, green apple, lemon, and ginger through a juicer.
- After juicing, thoroughly mix the ingredients.

Serve and enjoy:

- Pour the juice over ice for a refreshing finish.
- Garnish with a sprig of mint.

Nutritional Value (Approximate, Per Serving):

Calories: 80-100 kcal

Protein: 2-3g

Dietary Fibre: 4-6g

Vitamin A: 150-200% Daily Value

Vitamin C: 100-150% Daily Value

Iron: 2-3mg

Calcium: 50-80mg

Notes

Your

Observation

Citrus Burst Fibroid Fighter Juice

Ingredients:

- 2 oranges (peeled)
- 1 grapefruit (peeled)
- 1 carrot
- 1/2 beetroot
- 1-inch of turmeric root
- 1 tablespoon of chia seeds (soaked)

Preparation:

- Peel the oranges and grapefruits.
- Wash the carrot, beetroot, and turmeric root very well.
- Juice the oranges and grapefruit with a juicer.
- Run the carrot and beetroot through a juicer.
- Grate the turmeric root into the juice to enhance the flavour and health benefits.
- In a separate dish, soak chia seeds in water for a few minutes until they have a gel-like consistency.

- Add the soaked chia seeds to the juice.
- Stir well to combine all of the ingredients.

Serve and enjoy:

- Pour the juice into a glass and enjoy the citrusy blast.

Nutritional Value (Approximate, Per Serving):

Calories: 120-150 kcal

Protein: 3-4g

Dietary Fibre: 6-8g

Vitamin C: 200-250% Daily Value

Vitamin A: 80-100% Daily Value

Folate: 20-30% Daily Value

Iron: 2-3mg

Notes

Your

Observation

Ingredients:

- 2 cups of kale leaves (stems removed)
- 1 cucumber
- 1 green apple (cored and cut)
- 1 lemon (peeled)
- 1-inch piece of fresh ginger
- Handful of fresh mint leaves (optional)
- 1 celery stalk (optional)
- 1 cup of spinach leaves
- 1-2 cups of filtered water
- Ice cubes (optional)

Preparation:

- Wash all vegetables and fruits well.
- Cut the cucumber and green apple into manageable sizes.
- Peel the lemons and ginger.
- Combine the kale, cucumber, green apple, lemon, ginger, mint leaves (if using), and celery in a juicer.
- Juice the ingredients.

- Add the spinach leaves to the juicer and juice again.
- If the juice is excessively concentrated, dilute it with filtered water to your satisfaction.
- If you want a chilled cocktail, pour the juice over ice.

Nutritional Value (Approximate, Per Serving):

Calories: 70-90 kcal

Protein: 3-4g

Dietary Fibre: 5-7g

Vitamin A: 150-200% Daily Value

Vitamin C: 80-100% Daily Value

Iron: 2-3mg

Potassium: 500-600mg

Notes

Your
Observation

Cilantro-Cucumber Refresher

Ingredients:

- 1 cucumber
- Handful of fresh cilantro leaves
- 1 lime (juiced)
- 1-2 teaspoons of honey or agave syrup (optional for sweetness)
- 2 cups of cold water
- Ice cubes
- Sliced cucumber and cilantro for garnish (optional)

Preparation:

- Wash the cucumber and cilantro leaves very well.
- If the cucumber is not organic, peel it first and then slice it.
- Mix the cucumber slices, cilantro leaves, lime juice, and honey or agave syrup (if using) in a blender.
- Add cold water to the blender.
- Blend until it is smooth.

- Strain the mixture for a smoother consistency (optional).
- Refrigerate the combination for a short while or serve immediately over ice.
- If preferred, garnish with slices of cucumber and cilantro leaves.

Nutritional Value (Approximate, Per Serving):

Calories: 20-30 kcal

Carbohydrates: 5-7g

Sugars: 3-5g

Vitamin C: 20-30% Daily Value

Vitamin K: 30-40% Daily Value

Potassium: 150-200mg

Note

Your

Observation

Swiss Chard and Orange Infusion

Ingredients:

- 2 cups of Swiss chard leaves (stems removed)
- 2 oranges (peeled and segmented)
- 1 cucumber
- 1 lemon (peeled)
- 1-inch piece of ginger
- 1 tablespoon of flaxseeds (optional for extra nutrients)
- 1-2 cups of cold water
- Ice cubes (optional)

Preparation:

- Wash the Swiss chard leaves very well and remove the stems.
- If the cucumber is not organic, peel it first and then chop it into manageable pieces.
- Peel the oranges and lemons.

- Mix the Swiss chard leaves, orange segments, cucumber, lemon, ginger and flaxseeds (if using) in a juicer.
- Juice the ingredients.
- If the juice is excessively intense, dilute it with cold water to your satisfaction.
- Pour the juice over ice if desired.

Nutritional Value (Approximate, Per Serving):

Calories: 80-100 kcal

Protein: 3-4g

Dietary Fibre: 6-8g

Vitamin A: 150-180% Daily Value

Vitamin C: 120-150% Daily Value

Folate: 30-40% Daily Value

Potassium: 500-600mg

Notes

Your

Observation

Broccoli and Apple Vitality Juice

Ingredients:

- 2 cups of broccoli florets
- 2 green apples (cored and chopped)
- 1 cucumber
- 1 lemon (peeled)
- 1-inch piece of ginger
- 1-2 cups of cold water
- Ice cubes (optional)

Preparation:

- Wash the broccoli, apples, and cucumber very well.
- Cut the broccoli into tiny florets.
- Core and slice the apples.
- Peel the lemons and ginger.
- Combine broccoli florets, apple pieces, cucumber, lemon, and ginger in a juicer.
- Juice the ingredients.

- If the juice is excessively intense, dilute it with cold water to your satisfaction.
- Pour the juice over ice if desired.

Nutritional Value (Approximate, Per Serving):

Calories: 90-110 kcal

Protein: 3-4g

Dietary Fibre: 7-9g

Vitamin A: 20-30% Daily Value

Vitamin C: 150-180% Daily Value

Calcium: 80-100mg

Iron: 2-3mg

Notes

Your

Observation

Mustard Greens and Lemon Revitalizer

Ingredients:

- 2 cups of mustard greens (stems removed)
- 1 cucumber
- 1 green apple (cored and cut)
- 1 lemon (peeled)
- 1-inch piece of ginger
- 1-2 cups of cold water
- Ice cubes (optional)

Preparation:

- Wash the mustard greens well and remove the stems.
- Wash and chop the cucumber into manageable bits.
- Core and cut the green apple.
- Peel the lemons and ginger.
- Mix the mustard greens, cucumber, green apple, lemon, and ginger in a juicer.

- Juice the ingredients.
- If the juice is excessively intense, dilute it with cold water to your satisfaction.
- Pour the juice over ice if desired.

Nutritional Value (Approximate, Per Serving):

Calories: 70-90 kcal

Protein: 3-4g

Dietary Fibre: 6-8g

Vitamin A: 200-250% Daily Value

Vitamin C: 100-120% Daily Value

Folate: 30-40% Daily Value

Potassium: 500-600mg

Notes

Your

Observation

Arugula and Pineapple Bliss Juice

Ingredients:

- 2 cups of arugula
- 1 cup of pineapple chunks
- 1 cucumber
- 1 green apple (cored and cut)
- 1 lemon (peeled)
- 1-inch piece of ginger
- 1-2 cups of cold water
- Ice cubes (optional)

Preparation:

- Wash the arugula very well.
- Cut the cucumber and green apple into manageable pieces.
- Mix the arugula, pineapple pieces, cucumber, green apple, lemon and ginger in juicer.
- Juice the ingredients.
- If the juice is excessively intense, dilute it with cold water to your satisfaction.

- Pour the juice over ice if desired.

Nutritional Value (Approximate, Per Serving):

Calories: 80-100 kcal

Protein: 3-4g

Dietary Fibre: 6-8g

Vitamin A: 150-180% Daily Value

Vitamin C: 120-150% Daily Value

Folate: 20-30% Daily Value

Potassium: 400-500mg

Notes

Your

Observation

Beet Greens and Carrot Juice

Ingredients:

- 2 cups of beet greens (stems removed)
- 3 average-sized carrots
- 1 cucumber
- 1 green apple (cored and cut)
- 1 lemon (peeled)
- 1-inch piece of fresh ginger
- 1-2 cups of cold water
- Ice cubes (optional)

Preparation:

- Wash the beet greens very well and remove the stems.
- Wash the carrots and cucumbers, and chop them into manageable pieces.
- Core and slice the green apple.
- Peel the lemons and ginger.
- Mix beet greens, carrots, cucumber, green apple, lemon and ginger in a juicer.
- Juice the ingredients.

- If the juice is excessively concentrated, dilute it with cold water to your satisfaction.
- Pour the juice over ice if desired.

Nutritional Value (Approximate, Per Serving):

Calories: 80-100 kcal

Protein: 3-4g

Dietary Fibre: 6-8g

Vitamin A: 200-250% Daily Value

Vitamin C: 100-120% Daily Value

Folate: 30-40% Daily Value

Potassium: 500-600mg

Notes

Your

Observation

Watermelon Wonder Refresher

Ingredients:

- 2 cups of watermelon chunks (without seed)
- 1 cup of pineapple chunks
- 1/2 cup of strawberries (hulled)
- 1 lime, juiced
- Mint leaves for garnish (optional)
- Ice cubes (optional)

Preparation:

- Remove the seeds from the watermelon and chop into slices.
- Core and slice the pineapple.
- Hull the strawberries.
- Mix the watermelon, pineapple, strawberries, and lime juice in a blender.
- Blend until smooth.
- Strain the mixture for a smoother consistency (optional).

- Refrigerate the combination for a short while or serve immediately over ice.
- Garnish with mint leaves if desired.

Nutritional Value (Approximate, Per Serving):

Calories: 80-100 kcal

Carbohydrates: 20-25g

Sugars: 15-20g

Vitamin C: 80-100% Daily Value

Vitamin A: 20-30% Daily Value

Potassium: 200-300mg

Notes

Your

Observation

Apple Beet Bliss Juice

Ingredients:

- 2 average-sized apples (any sweet variety)
- 1 average-sized beetroot (peeled and sliced)
- 1 cucumber
- 1/2 lemon, juiced
- 1-inch piece of ginger
- 1-2 cups of cold water
- Ice cubes (optional)

Preparation:

- Wash and core the apples well.
- Peel and slice the beetroot.
- Wash and chop the cucumber into manageable pieces.
- Juice the apples, beetroot, cucumber, lemon juice, and ginger using a juicer.
- If the juice is too concentrated, dilute it with cold water according to your preference.

- Pour the juice over ice if desired.

Nutritional Value (Approximate, Per Serving):

Calories: 90-110 kcal

Protein: 2-3g

Dietary Fibre: 4-6g

Vitamin C: 30-40% Daily Value

Iron: 1-2mg

Folate: 20-30% Daily Value

Potassium: 300-400mg

Notes

Your

Observation

Dandelion Greens and Carrot Crush Juice

Ingredients:

- 2 cups of dandelion greens (stems removed)
- 4 average-sized carrots
- 1 cucumber
- 1 green apple (cored and sliced)
- 1 lemon (peeled)
- 1-inch piece of ginger
- 1-2 cups of cold water
- Ice cubes (optional)

Preparation:

- Wash the dandelion greens very well and remove the stems.
- Wash and peel the carrots. Cut them into manageable bits.
- Wash and chop the cucumber into bits.
- Core and slice the green apple.
- Peel the lemons and ginger.

- Mix the dandelion greens, carrots, cucumber, green apple, lemon, and ginger in a juicer.
- Juice the ingredients.
- If the juice is excessively intense, dilute it with cold water to your satisfaction.
- Pour the juice over ice if desired.

Nutritional Value (Approximate, Per Serving):

Calories: 80-100 kcal

Protein: 3-4g

Dietary Fibre: 6-8g

Vitamin A: 300-350% Daily Value

Vitamin C: 80-100% Daily Value

Folate: 30-40% Daily Value

Potassium: 500-600mg

Notes

Your
Observation

Watercress and Grapefruit Zest Juice

Ingredients:

- 2 cups of watercress (stems removed)
- 2 pink of grapefruits (peeled and segmented)
- 1 cucumber
- 1 green apple (cored and cut)
- 1 lime, juiced
- 1-inch piece of ginger
- 1-2 cups of cold water
- Ice cubes (optional)

Preparation:

- Wash watercress very well and remove the stems.
- Peel and segment the grapefruits.
- Wash and chop the cucumber into manageable pieces.
- Core and cut the green apple.

- Combine watercress, grapefruit segments, cucumber, green apple, lime juice, and ginger in a juicer.
- Juice the ingredients.
- If the juice is excessively intense, dilute it with cold water to your satisfaction.
- Pour the juice over ice if desired.

Nutritional Value (Approximate, Per Serving):

Calories: 70-90 kcal

Protein: 2-3g

Dietary Fibre: 4-6g

Vitamin A: 150-180% Daily Value

Vitamin C: 120-150% Daily Value

Folate: 30-40% Daily Value

Potassium: 400-500mg

Notes

Your

Observation

Red Zinger Juice

Ingredients:

- 1 average-sized beetroot (peeled and cut)
- 1 cup of strawberries (hulled)
- 1/2 cup of raspberries
- 1/2 cup of blueberries
- 1 cucumber
- 1 lime, juiced
- 1-inch piece of ginger
- 1-2 cups of cold water
- Ice cubes (optional)

Preparation:

- Peel and slice the beetroot.
- Hull the strawberries.
- Combine the beetroot pieces, strawberries, raspberries, blueberries, cucumber, lime juice, and ginger in a blender.
- If you want your juice cooler, add some ice cubes.
- Blend until smooth.

- Strain the mixture for a smoother consistency (optional).
- Dilute the juice with cold water according to your taste.
- Pour the juice over ice if desired.

Nutritional Value (Approximate, Per Serving):

Calories: 80-100 kcal

Protein: 2-3g

Dietary Fibre: 5-7g

Vitamin C: 80-100% Daily Value

Folate: 20-30% Daily Value

Potassium: 300-400mg

Notes

Your

Observation

Cucumber Spinach Refresher

Ingredients:

- 1 cucumber
- 2 cups of fresh spinach leaves
- 1 green apple (cored and cut)
- 1 lemon (peeled)
- 1-inch piece of ginger
- 1-2 cups of cold water
- Ice cubes (optional)

Preparation:

- Wash the cucumber, spinach leaves, and green apple very well.
- Cut the cucumber and green apple into manageable pieces.
- Peel the lemons and ginger.
- Mix cucumber, spinach leaves, green apple, lemon, and ginger in a juicer.
- Juice the ingredients.
- If the juice is excessively concentrated, dilute it with cold water to your satisfaction.

- Pour the juice over ice if desired.

Nutritional Value (Approximate, Per Serving):

Calories: 60-80 kcal

Protein: 2-3g

Dietary Fiber: 4-6g

Vitamin A: 150-180% Daily Value

Vitamin C: 80-100% Daily Value

Folate: 40-50% Daily Value

Potassium: 300-400mg

Notes

Your

Observation

Spinach Celery Vitality Juice

Ingredients:

- 2 cups of fresh spinach leaves
- 4 celery stalks
- 1 cucumber
- 1 green apple (cored and cut)
- 1/2 lemon, juiced
- 1-inch piece of ginger
- 1-2 cups of cold water
- Ice cubes (optional)

Preparation:

- Wash the spinach, celery stalks, and cucumber well.
- Slice the celery and cucumber into manageable bits.
- Core and cut the green apple.
- Combine fresh spinach, celery, cucumber, green apple, lemon juice, and ginger in a juicer.
- Juice the ingredients.

- If the juice is excessively intense, dilute it with cold water to your satisfaction.
- Pour the juice over ice if desired.

Nutritional Value (Approximate, Per Serving):

Calories: 60-80 kcal

Protein: 3-4g

Dietary Fibre: 4-6g

Vitamin A: 150-180% Daily Value

Vitamin C: 80-100% Daily Value

Folate: 40-50% Daily Value

Potassium: 400-500mg

Notes

Your
Observation

CHAPTER 4: SMOOTHIE RECIPES FOR FIBROID

Pineapple Turmeric Power Smoothie

Ingredients:

- 1 cup of pineapple chunks
- 1 banana
- 1/2 teaspoon of turmeric powder (or 1-inch of turmeric root, fresh and peeled)
- 1 tablespoon of chia seeds
- 1 cup of leafy greens (spinach or kale)
- 1/2 cup of Greek yogurt (optional for creaminess)
- 1 cup of coconut water or almond milk
- Ice cubes (optional)

Preparation:

- Peel and slice the banana.
- If using fresh turmeric root, peel it and cut it into smaller pieces.

- Combine the pineapple, banana, turmeric, chia seeds, leafy greens, and Greek yoghurt (if using) in a blender.
- Pour in the coconut water or almond milk.
- If you want your smoothie cooler, add ice cubes.
- Blend until smooth and creamy.
- If necessary, increase the liquid content to get the desired consistency.

Serve and enjoy:

- Pour into a glass and enjoy the revitalising Pineapple Turmeric Power Smoothie.

Nutritional Value (Approximate, Per Serving):

Calories: 250-300 kcal

Protein: 8-10g

Dietary Fibre: 7-9g

Vitamin C: 100-120% Daily Value

Vitamin K: 60-80% Daily Value

Manganese: 40-50% Daily Value

Potassium: 600-700mg

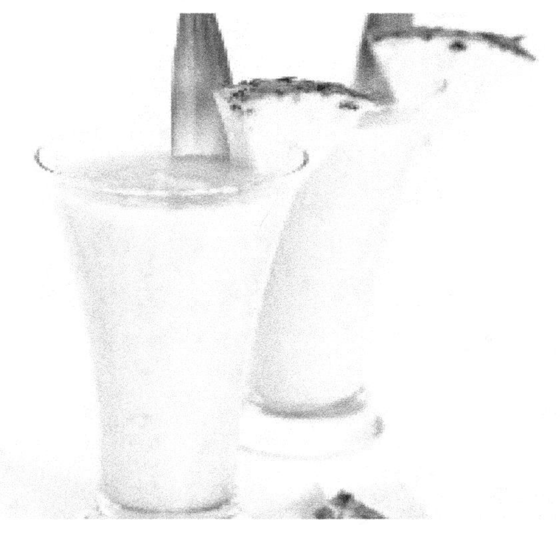

Notes

Your

Observation

Kale and Berry Blast Smoothie

Ingredients:

- 1 cup kale leaves (stems removed)
- 1/2 cup of blueberries
- 1/2 cup of strawberries (hulled)
- 1/2 cup of raspberries
- 1 banana
- 1 tablespoon of chia seeds
- 1 cup of almond milk or coconut water
- Ice cubes (optional)

Preparation:

- Wash the kale leaves very well and remove the stems.
- Rinse the berries with cool water.
- Peel and slice the banana.
- Mix the kale, blueberries, strawberries, raspberries, banana, and chia seeds in a blender.
- Pour in the almond milk or coconut water.

- If you like a cooler consistency, add some ice cubes.
- Blend until smooth and creamy.
- If required, add more liquid to get the desired thickness.

Serve and enjoy:

- Pour the colourful Kale and Berry Blast Smoothie into a glass.

Nutritional Value (Approximate, Per Serving):

Calories: 150-180 kcal

Protein: 4-5g

Dietary Fibre: 8-10g

Vitamin C: 80-100% Daily Value

Vitamin K: 200-250% Daily Value

Folate: 40-50% Daily Value

Potassium: 400-500mg

Notes

Your

Observation

Cucumber Mint Refresher

Ingredients:

- 1 cucumber
- Handful of fresh mint leaves
- 1 lime, juiced
- 1 tablespoon of honey or agave syrup (optional)
- 2 cups of cold water
- Ice cubes
- Sliced cucumber and mint for garnish (optional)

Preparation:

- Wash the cucumber very well and peel if it is not organic.
- Cut the cucumber into slices.
- In a blender, mix cucumber slices and fresh mint leaves.
- Squeeze the lime juice into the blender.
- For a sweeter flavour, add honey or agave syrup (optional).
- Pour in cold water.
- Blend until it is smooth.

- To remove pulp (optional), strain the mixture through a fine mesh screen.
- Refrigerate the combination for a short while or serve immediately over ice.
- Garnish with cucumber slices and mint leaves if preferred.

Nutritional Value (Approximate, Per Serving):

Calories: 20-30 kcal

Carbohydrates: 5-7g

Sugars: 3-5g

Vitamin C: 20-30% Daily Value

Vitamin K: 30-40% Daily Value

Potassium: 150-200mg

Notes

Your

Observation

Collard Greens and Pineapple Paradise Smoothie

Ingredients:

- 2 cups of collard greens (stems removed)
- 1 cup of pineapple chunks
- 1 banana
- 1/2 lime (juiced)
- 1-inch piece of fresh ginger
- 1 tablespoon of chia seeds
- 1 cup of coconut water
- Ice cubes (optional)

Preparation:

- Wash the collard greens very well and remove the stems.
- Peel and slice a banana.
- Juice a lime.
- Mix the collard greens, pineapple chunks, banana, lime juice, fresh

ginger, chia seeds, and coconut water in a blender.

- If you want your smoothie cooler, add ice cubes.
- Blend until smooth and creamy.
- If required, add additional coconut water to get the desired thickness.
- Pour into a glass and savour the tropical paradise.

Nutritional Value (Approximate, Per Serving):

Calories: 180-220 kcal

Protein: 5-6g

Dietary Fibre: 8-10g

Vitamin A: 200-250% Daily Value

Vitamin C: 150-180% Daily Value

Calcium: 150-180mg

Iron: 2-3mg

Notes

Your

Observation

Spinach Surprise Smoothie

Ingredients:

- 2 cups of fresh spinach leaves
- 1 banana
- 1/2 cup of pineapple chunks
- 1/2 cup of mango chunks
- 1/2 cucumber
- 1 tablespoon of chia seeds
- 1 cup of coconut water or almond milk
- Ice cubes (optional)

Preparation:

- Wash the spinach leaves very well.
- Peel and slice the banana.
- Combine fresh spinach, banana, pineapple, mango, cucumber, chia seeds, and coconut water or almond milk in a blender.
- If you want your smoothie cooler, add ice cubes.
- Blend until smooth and creamy.

- If necessary, increase the liquid content to get the desired consistency.
- Pour into a glass and enjoy the nutrient-rich Spinach Surprise Smoothie.

Nutritional Value (Approximate, Per Serving):

Calories: 250-300 kcal

Protein: 8-10g

Dietary Fibre: 7-9g

Vitamin C: 150-180% Daily Value

Vitamin K: 200-250% Daily Value

Folate: 40-50% Daily Value

Potassium: 600-700mg

Notes

Your

Observation

Tropical Tango Smoothie

Ingredients:

- 1 cup of pineapple chunks
- 1/2 cup of mango chunks
- 1/2 cup of papaya chunks
- 1 banana
- 1/2 cup of Greek yogurt (optional for creaminess)
- 1 tablespoon of flaxseeds
- 1/2 lime, juiced
- 1 cup of coconut water or pineapple juice
- Ice cubes (optional)

Preparation:

- Peel and chop pineapple, mango, and papaya into pieces.
- Peel the banana.
- Mix the pineapple, mango, papaya, banana, Greek yoghurt (if using), flaxseeds, lime juice, and coconut water or pineapple juice in a blender.

- If you want your smoothie cooler, add ice cubes.
- Blend until smooth and creamy.
- If necessary, increase the liquid content to get the desired consistency.
- Pour into a glass and enjoy the Tropical Tango Smoothie.

Nutritional Value (Approximate, Per Serving):

Calories: 250-300 kcal

Protein: 8-10g

Dietary Fibre: 7-9g

Vitamin C: 150-180% Daily Value

Vitamin A: 80-100% Daily Value

Folate: 30-40% Daily Value

Potassium: 600-700mg

Notes

Your

Observation

Berry Bliss Anti-Inflammatory Smoothie

Ingredients:

- 1 cup of mixed berries (blueberries, strawberries, raspberries)
- 1 banana
- 1/2 cup of pineapple chunks
- 1 tablespoon of flaxseeds
- 1 cup of leafy greens (spinach or kale)
- 1 cup of coconut water

Preparation:

- Rinse the berries and leafy leave very well.
- Peel and slice the banana.
- Mix berries, banana, pineapple pieces, flaxseeds, and leafy greens in a blender.
- Pour in the coconut water.
- Blend until smooth and creamy.
- If necessary, add additional coconut water to get the required consistency.

Serve and enjoy:

- Pour into a glass and savour the berry-infused sweetness.

Nutritional Value (Approximate, Per Serving):

Calories: 200-250 kcal

Protein: 4-5g

Dietary Fibre: 8-10g

Vitamin C: 150-200% Daily Value

Vitamin K: 80-100% Daily Value

Manganese: 30-40% Daily Value

Omega-3 Fatty Acids from Flaxseeds: 1-2g

Notes

Your

Observation

Ingredients:

- 2 cups of fresh spinach leaves
- 2 ripe pears (cored and cut)
- 1 banana
- 1/2 cup of Greek yogurt (optional for creaminess)
- 1 tablespoon of chia seeds
- 1/2 lemon, juiced
- 1-inch piece of ginger
- 1-2 cups of cold water
- Ice cubes (optional)

Preparation:

- Rinse the spinach leaves completely.
- Core and slice the ripe pears.
- Peel a banana.
- Combine the fresh spinach, cut pears, banana, Greek yoghurt (if using), chia seeds, lemon juice, and ginger in a blender.

- If you want your smoothie cooler, add ice cubes.
- Blend until smooth and creamy.
- If necessary, increase the liquid content to get the desired consistency.
- Pour into a glass and enjoy the Spinach-Pear Dream Smoothie.

Nutritional Value (Approximate, Per Serving):

Calories: 250-300 kcal

Protein: 8-10g

Dietary Fiber: 7-9g

Vitamin C: 30-40% Daily Value

Vitamin K: 200-250% Daily Value

Folate: 40-50% Daily Value

Potassium: 600-700mg

Notes

Your

Observation

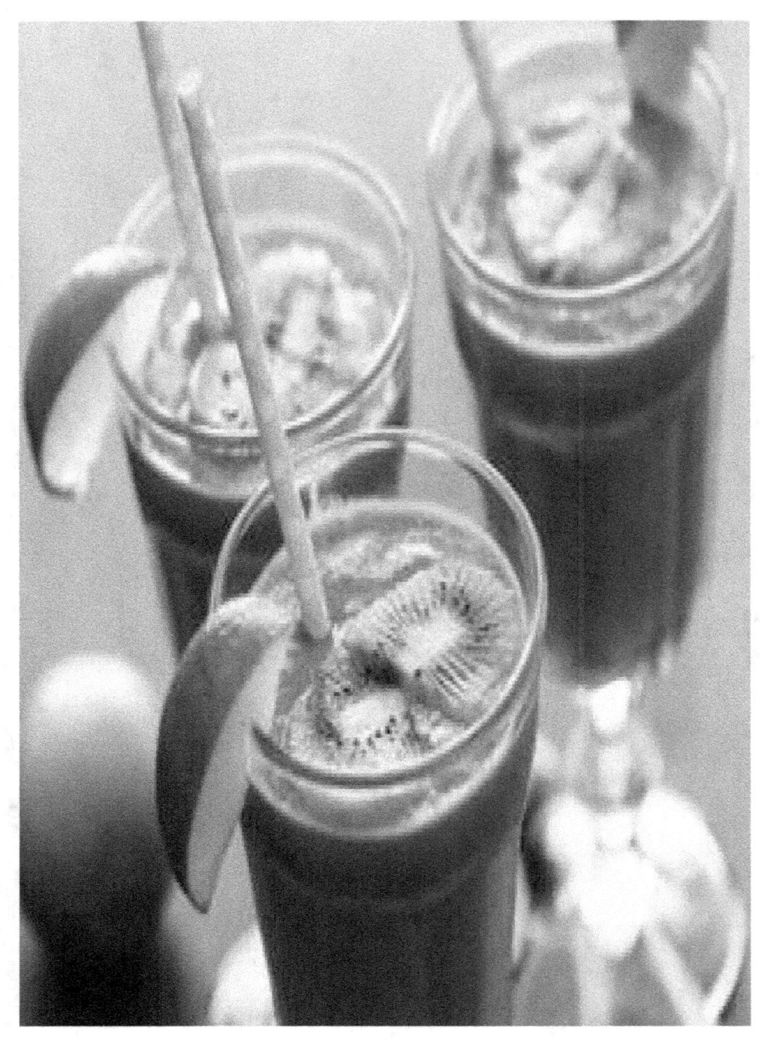

CHAPTER 5

Incorporating Therapeutic Herbs for Fibroid Health

When addressing fibroid control through nutrition, the use of soothing herbs can provide an added layer of assistance. These herbs not only improve the flavour of your juices and smoothies, but they also have medicinal characteristics that may benefit your general health. Here are some therapeutic herbs to consider include in your fibroid-friendly recipes.

Ginger:

Properties: Anti-inflammatory and anti-nausea.

Incorporation: Add a tiny piece of fresh ginger to drinks or smoothies for a spicy bite.

Turmeric:

Properties: potent anti-inflammatory and antioxidant.

To reap the therapeutic effects of turmeric, mix it into smoothies or drinks with either powder or raw root.

Mint:

Properties: Soothing for digestion and refreshing.

Incorporation: Sprinkle fresh mint leaves into your liquids for a blast of flavour and probable digestive aid.

Dandelions:

Properties: detoxifying, high in vitamins and minerals.

Incorporation: Add dandelion greens to green juices or smoothies for a slight bitterness and extra nutrients.

Cinnamon:

Properties: Anti-inflammatory; may help manage blood sugar.

Incorporation: Add a sprinkle of cinnamon to your smoothies for warmth and probable health benefits.

Red Clover:

Properties: Historically used to regulate hormones.

Incorporation: Make red clover tea and use it as a basis for your smoothies.

Milk thistle:

Properties: Liver-supportive and antioxidant.

Incorporation: Make milk thistle tea and use it as a basis, or use milk thistle extract into your dishes.

Rosemary:

Properties: Anti-inflammatory, high in antioxidants.

Incorporation: Infuse rosemary into water or add a little bit to drinks and smoothies.

Nettle:

Properties: Nutritious, typically used for menstruation support.

Incorporation: Steep nettle tea and use it as a foundation for drinks.

Basil:

Properties: anti-inflammatory, high in vitamins.

Incorporate: Put a few fresh basil leaves into your smoothies for a distinct flavour profile.

Experiment with these medicinal herbs to find combinations that not only satisfy your taste senses but also support your fibroid control aims. Always speak with a healthcare practitioner, especially if you have specific health problems or are taking drugs, since herbs can interact with some pharmaceuticals.

CHAPTER 6: LIFESTYLE CHANGES FOR FIBROID MANAGEMENT

Lifestyle adjustments can help manage fibroids and alleviate their symptoms. While these modifications may not remove fibroids, they can improve general health and help manage symptoms. Here are some lifestyle changes to consider for fibroid control:

Maintain a healthy diet:

Promote a diet high in fruits, vegetables, whole grains, and lean proteins.

Include iron-rich meals to avoid anaemia, which can be connected with excessive menstrual flow.

Consider consuming anti-inflammatory foods like fatty fish, nuts, seeds, and leafy greens.

Manage Weight:

Maintain a healthy weight by exercising regularly and eating a balanced diet.

Obesity has been related to an increased risk of fibroids, which can worsen symptoms.

Exercise regularly:

Regular physical activity can help control weight and reduce stress.

Moderate exercise, such as brisk walking, swimming, or yoga, is good.

Stay hydrated:

Drink enough of water to maintain your overall health and hydration.

Manage stress:

Use stress-reduction practices such as meditation, deep breathing, and yoga.

Chronic stress may cause hormonal abnormalities, which might affect fibroid development.

Adequate Sleep:

Aim for 7-9 hours of good sleep every night.

Adequate sleep promotes hormonal balance and immune function, which can improve fibroid management.

Lack of sleep has been linked to increased stress and hormonal abnormalities, which may influence fibroid development.

Limit Caffeine and Alcohol:

Caffeine should be consumed in moderation, since excessive consumption may raise the risk of fibroids.

Limit your alcohol consumption since too much alcohol might disrupt hormonal balance.

Quit smoking:

Smoking has been linked to an increased chance of developing fibroids, and it may exacerbate symptoms.

Consider Hormone-Healthy Habits:

Investigate hormone-healthy habits such as frequent, moderate exercise and keeping a healthy weight.

Avoid using hormonal contraception or hormone replacement treatment without medical supervision.

Regular Check-Ups:

Attend frequent gynaecological check-ups to evaluate fibroid development and symptoms.

Discuss treatment choices and management techniques with your healthcare practitioner.

Explore Complementary Therapies:

Some people get comfort from alternative therapies such as acupuncture, chiropractic care, and herbal supplements.

Before considering any alternative remedies, consult with a healthcare practitioner.

It is critical to remember that lifestyle modifications should be discussed with your healthcare professional, and personalised treatment regimens should be developed for your unique circumstance. Fibroids vary in size and symptoms, and a healthcare expert may advise you on the best management techniques for your specific situation.

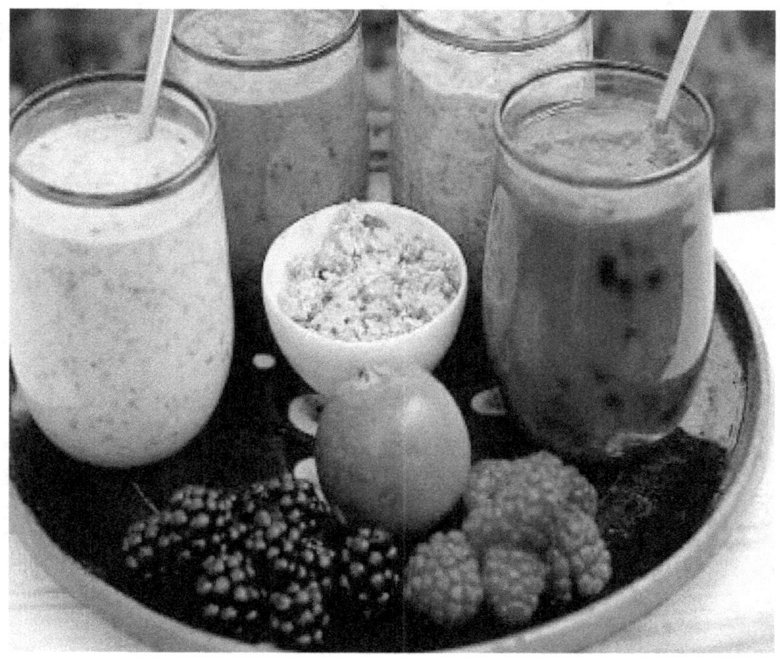

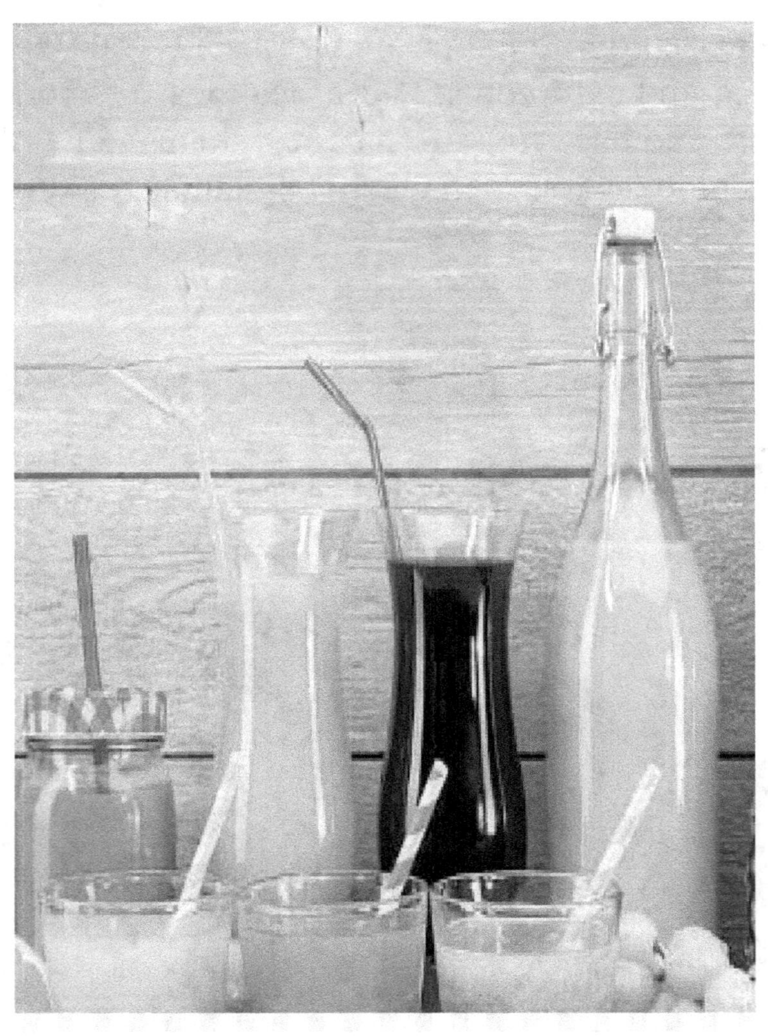

CHAPTER 7: CONCLUSION

Finally, integrating juicing and smoothies into a fibroid control diet provides a tasty and nutritious technique that promotes overall health and wellness. Fruits, vegetables, and other fibroid-friendly items can supply critical vitamins, minerals, and antioxidants while also increasing hydration levels. These beverages provide not only a delightful alternative to typical meals, but also a practical way to get fibroid-specific nutrients into the diet.

Individuals may actively contribute to their general health by concentrating on substances with possible fibroid control advantages, such as leafy greens, berries, and anti-inflammatory components. Furthermore, hydrating and nutrient-dense concoctions can help you maintain a healthy weight, balance your hormones, and manage fibroids-related symptoms.

Juicing and smoothies should be used as part of a complete strategy to fibroid control, including other lifestyle modifications like as a good diet, frequent exercise, stress management, and adequate sleep. Consulting with a healthcare physician is vital for tailoring these dietary recommendations to individual needs and ensuring they are consistent with a successful, personalised fibroid management strategy. Individuals who commit to mindful diet and a holistic lifestyle can empower themselves on their quest to fibroid control and improved overall well-being.

STAY HEALTHY!

www.ingramcontent.com/pod-product-compliance
Lightning Source LLC
Chambersburg PA
CBHW070824260726
48660CB00005B/1974